The Five Finger Lifestyle Diet

The Five Finger Lifestyle Diet

Dan Eichenbaum, MD

To order additional copies of this book, contact:
Xlibris Corporation
1-888-795-4274
www.Xlibris.com
Orders@Xlibris.com
64220

Contents

If you are overweight and you want to lose excess pounds to improve your health and physical appearance . . .

If you are diabetic with poorly controlled blood sugars and you are determined to take charge of your disease, reduce your blood sugar to the normal range, and try to prevent the debilitating and disabling complications of diabetes . . .

There are five foods that you cannot eat:

1. Bread and baked goods
2. Potatoes and other root vegetables
3. Rice
4. Pasta
5. Fruit except for berries

That is my Five-Finger Lifestyle.

The rest of this book is just commentary.

Introduction

For most of my life, as a child and a young adult, I was skinny. In fact, I was so skinny that I could disappear by turning sideways. In my preschool years, I was cared for by my mother's mother while my parents worked. As with any doting grandmother (I was the first grandchild), part of her mission was to be sure I ate enough. In those days (and more so today), evidence of sufficient feeding was a chubby laughing baby. Unfortunately, I was a picky eater, and my parents and grandmother had to find ingenious ways to get me to eat. I remember mashed-potato airplanes flying toward my mouth and "choo-choo train" vegetables making their way along my plate. When my parents weren't there, my grandmother laboriously prepared multiple main courses for each meal. After taking a bite or two, I would ask her to make something different. A willing enabler, eager to do her job, my grandmother always complied with my request.

When I was four years old, we moved into our own home. Both my parents worked full time as pediatric dentists, but we had home-cooked dinner every night. My mother prepared oven-ready meals late at night or in the early morning, and they were delicious. Best of all, we always had dessert. My mother could really bake, and dessert usually consisted of cake with frosting. Ice cream was also involved. Freshly baked chocolate chip cookies were prepared and available for twenty-four-hour snacking.

As dentists, my parents did not allow candy in the house. To this day, I have little craving for candy bars. When it comes to cakes and cookies, however, saying "no, thank you" is much more difficult than eating "mass quantities."

Gradually, I expanded my food repertoire. By college, I was eating a normal "collegiate" diet, which consisted primarily of cheeseburgers, french fries, and chocolate milk shakes. By medical school, I expanded my diet to include other ethnic cuisines. I learned to appreciate and prepare Chinese, Indonesian, Indian, French, German, and Mexican foods. Cookies and cakes, my sweet addictions, remained a constant part of my daily eating regimen.

My weight remained fairly constant all those years. I was thin and healthy, participated in sports, and ate whatever I wanted. After graduating from medical school, however, my weight slowly started to increase. Over the next thirty years, I gained about 70 pounds without even knowing it. It was as if I suddenly woke up one morning and weighed in at 225 pounds with a total cholesterol of 230. Unbelievable!

Eating habits are formed at an early age. The foods that we eat as children are associated with satisfaction and comfort, which is why they are commonly called comfort foods. Since children have little or no independent ability to make food choices for themselves, the cuisine parents feed their kids determines a child's weight and future food choices. To this day, when I make a Hungarian-style beef stew, I can picture myself sitting at the dinner table in my paternal grandparents' apartment. It is no wonder that, as adults, it is difficult to break these childhood eating habits.

In my own case, with a strong family history of diabetes, hypertension, and stroke, I knew that I was heading down a dangerous path. I took action by actually going to an internist for care. He considered my family history and suggested that I try a low-carbohydrate diet. Although skeptical at first, I took his advice. Nine years later, I am still successfully living low carb.

I have taken the time to tell you these facts about my own personal eating history to illustrate some basic principles that define most of our eating habits. Also, I wanted you to understand that I prescribe the low-carbohydrate lifestyle to my patients and to you because it worked so well for me.

Face it. Sugar and carbohydrates taste great! That's why it is so difficult for us to stop eating them.

And that is why I wrote this book.

My goal is to give you a simple, understandable eating lifestyle to break the carbohydrate addiction that will ruin your health and shorten your life.

Most of you will easily recognize that the Five-Finger Lifestyle promotes the same low-carbohydrate dietary regimen originally proposed by Robert C. Atkins, MD, in 1972. His first book, *Dr. Atkins' Diet Revolution*, was a true ideological revolution. For years, the food industry—through its governmental, dietary, and medical accomplices—had promoted a low-calorie, low-fat diet regimen. The "taboo" list included eggs, butter, cheese, beef, pork, creamy sauces, ice cream, and anything intrinsically delicious or prepared in a delicious manner. We were allowed to eat chicken, fish, fruit, nothing fried, and a variety of veggies best identified as rabbit food. Snacks, especially those that were commercially available, had to contain high amounts of carbohydrates to make up for the excluded eggs, cream, and butter needed for the product to taste good.

Peer pressure and guilt were also an integral part of the low-fat, low-calorie program. Imagine going out to dinner with friends. They all order dry, grilled chicken breast, baked potato (margarine only, please), and garden salad with fat-free dressing. You turn yourself into the evening's pariah by ordering a steak with béarnaise sauce, a bacon cheeseburger, or a rack of baby back ribs. While you are sitting there trying to enjoy your delicious meal, you are the subject of criticism and scorn, and it is suggested that they will be happy to take you directly to the emergency room after the meal.

Trust me. I have been there!

Dr. Atkins's approach contradicted those accepted rules. He recognized that the twin epidemics of obesity and adult-onset diabetes were the result of a national diet high in carbohydrates. Based on sound physiology, medical evidence, and clinical success, he tried to change the dietary regimen of the country. Unfortunately, he was bucking a strong, well-financed campaign to maintain the status quo. In a series of books published over the ensuing thirty years, Dr. Atkins carefully outlined and explained the benefits of the low-carbohydrate diet.

Let me assure you that I am a disciple of Dr. Atkins. I agree with his approach to weight and sugar control. In fact, I urge all of you to read his books to get a more complete discussion of carbohydrate restriction. His chapters about specific carbohydrate content of various foods and how to estimate portion size are important in order to follow a low-carbohydrate regimen successfully.

Legitimately, you could ask me why I decided to write this book.

Simply put, thirty years after Dr. Atkins's first book, Americans continue to gain weight and develop adult-onset diabetes at an alarming rate. The costs of this epidemic—in terms of death, disability, and essential medical/ nursing care—are enormous and continuing to increase. Each of us, directly or indirectly, is paying the price through obesity, diabetes, disease, increased insurance premiums, and higher taxes.

Nevertheless, establishment diet "gurus" and government "nannies" continue to push low-calorie, low-fat, portion-controlled eating regimens that are plainly too complex and require too much willpower for average people to follow. In addition, most of the time, they just don't work.

Consider this book an instruction manual for eating, a how-to book for managing food intake, and a catechism to help you live a healthy lifestyle.

The Five-Finger Lifestyle
The Untouchables

The first part of living the Five-Finger Lifestyle is to understand what foods you may *not* eat and why they are not good for you.

Bread and baked goods

Most bread and baked goods are made primarily from flour and sugar. In carbohydrate-content terms, a quarter cup of all-purpose flour contains 20 grams of carbohydrates, and a teaspoon of sugar contains 4 grams. Whether made from scratch in your kitchen, from a prepackaged mix, or purchased already baked and wrapped in cellophane, these items are filled with carbohydrates. If you are talented enough to bake at home, you can control the final carbohydrate content to a certain degree. The flour and sugar origin of baked goods, however, guarantees that the carb content will be too high. Baked goods that are manufactured often have additives that further increase the carb content, usually to enhance the sweetness of the final product. It is not unusual for store-bought bread to have 24-40 grams of carbs per slice. Certain products like bagels contain well over 40 grams of carbs due to their density. And when it comes to the sweet stuff like doughnuts, pastries, cakes, and pies, the added glazes, fruits, toppings, frostings, and sugars send the carb content through the roof.

Bread and baked goods are such a common part of our diet that avoiding them is really difficult. These are foods we all eat routinely and without thinking. For example, a simple sandwich with two slices of bread, a lunchtime staple, starts you off with 50 grams of carbohydrates before you add anything else. Include a banana or a slice of pie, and your total climbs well over 100 grams. Many snack items also fall into this category. Pretzels, crackers, cookies, and a variety of packaged treats are readily available and all bad.

Potatoes and root vegetables

When the part of the plant we eat is the plant's root, it is called a root vegetable. A root vegetable stores carbohydrate in its root for later use. The green leafy part above the ground manufactures carbohydrates using energy from the sun. Most root vegetables are high in carbohydrate content. Commonly eaten vegetables in this category are potatoes, sweet potatoes, beets, carrots, taro, and other various tubers.

Would you like fries with that?

Rice

Rice contains lots of carbohydrates. Again, the part of the plant we eat is the part where carbohydrate is stored. Generally, there is between 34 and 45 grams of carbohydrate in only one-quarter cup of uncooked white or brown rice. That "standard" portion (1/4 cup) is ridiculously small compared to the "normal" portion that most people eat at a meal. Eating rice raises blood sugar both because it is high in carbohydrates as a food and because the amount generally eaten at a single meal far exceeds the ridiculously miniscule "single portion" used for carb comparison purposes.

Pasta

Pasta is made almost entirely from flour. As such, it has a very high carbohydrate content per quarter-cup serving (about 45 grams). When was the last time you saw a quarter-cup serving of pasta at a meal? Pasta is, unfortunately, another high-carbohydrate food that is eaten in large quantities.

Fruit except for berries

Because fruits are natural, we have been conditioned to believe that eating fruit is part of a healthy lifestyle. In truth, from a carbohydrate perspective, fruit is a big sac of sugar around some seeds. Bananas, citrus fruits, and melons are particularly high in carbohydrates. Remember, just because these sugars are natural, they are still carbohydrates and, therefore, will raise your blood sugar.

Those are the foods you cannot eat—the five fingers of my Five-Finger Lifestyle. Learning which foods fall into each category and *avoiding* them form the basis for this very simple method you can use to lose weight and control your blood sugar. Just saying *no* to these items results in weight loss and lower blood sugar levels and gets you started on the right track.

In addition, there are food items you should know are bad for you. I mean, you should know instinctively that you cannot eat them.

Let's call these the *miscellaneous untouchable items of the obvious kind*:

1. Candy of all kinds, even on Valentine's Day (okay, maybe one piece on that day)
2. Nondiet sodas, soft drinks, or energy drinks
3. Sugar (yes, even natural raw or organic sugar)
4. Sweet tea unless sweetened with Splenda
5. Honey-roasted anything
6. Most breakfast cereals and grits
7. Breakfast or energy bars that are high in carbohydrates
8. Oreos and Twinkies (these items deserve a separate category)
9. Cakes, pies, cookies, sweet snacks, chips, etc.

That's it, at least what you cannot eat.

The simple part is that you don't have to weigh, measure, compare, exchange, look up, or keep track of anything. You do have to think. You also have to have some willpower. And you do have to understand what food falls into which category.

After you understand what you *can* eat, you will begin to see that you can be successful and still be gastronomically satisfied.

Read on!

The Five-Finger Lifestyle
Basic Concepts

So now that you know what foods to avoid, let's talk about what you can and do eat.

To live the Five-Finger Lifestyle, you are going to replace all those forbidden carbohydrates with protein and fat. Protein becomes your primary staple. The fats that you eat are more incidental; that is, they come along with the protein or are used in the preparation of the protein you eat. Remember, you are changing your metabolism from carbohydrate-burning to fat-burning mode. That is why this regimen is so successful.

Animals provide our main source of protein. You can eat all forms of meat and fish. You can also eat eggs and dairy products. All of these foods are reliable protein sources. It is easy to imagine yourself eating a char-grilled steak, blackened fish, sautéed shrimp, or roasted pork. Of course, these meals may seem too complex for your kitchen skills. Like many things in life, however, there are tricks you can use to make these delicious meals and many more with a little advance preparation and minimal effort.

When it comes to everyday meals, eating protein instead of carbohydrates is easier than you would think. As a society, we have become accustomed to eating quickly, grabbing a meal on the go. This accounts for the popularity of finger foods, fast foods, and the ubiquitous sandwich. The sandwich is the ultimate finger food—an entire meal between two pieces of bread.

All it takes to eliminate the sandwich is a little innovation combined with a knife and fork. Let's say you want to eat a cheeseburger for lunch. Put the burger on a plate, top it off with cheese and whatever other toppings you want (onions, pickles, tomatoes, etc.), and eat it with a knife and fork. A tuna melt tastes almost as good on a plate without the bread, especially when you realize how good you will look and feel when you lose all that extra weight. Arrange the tuna salad on your plate, melt cheese over it in the microwave, and eat it with a knife and fork. Luncheon meat and cheese can be rolled together and eaten as finger food or arranged on a plate with condiments.

Most of the sandwiches you eat for quick meals are easily converted to knife-and-fork fare on a plate. One unexpected benefit of eliminating the sandwich could be sitting down to eat, a truly relaxing event, a brief moment of sanity in an otherwise hectic day. For those who just cannot sit down to eat, a variety of low-carb wraps are available. That is a good compromise for the time-challenged individual. Just be sure that what is inside the wrap falls into the acceptable category.

Of course, the best strategy is to make your lunch at home and bring it with you. The lunch box used to be part of everyone's normal daily routine. It still is the best way to control the quality, quantity, and content of your meals.

Tips to help you succeed

The Five-Finger Lifestyle is not a prescription for a life of hunger. Hunger is caused by low blood sugar. Eating a carbohydrate load triggers a rapid increase in blood insulin level, which quickly lowers blood sugar. Limiting carbohydrate intake, therefore, will cause a general decrease in hunger. The longer you follow the Five-Finger Lifestyle, the less food craving you will feel.

Another benefit of carbohydrate restriction is that portion control is not strictly required as long as you follow the program guidelines. I do encourage you, however, to exercise reasonable restraint on how much you eat at each meal. One successful strategy to limit quantity and to conquer your hunger is to eat multiple small meals throughout the day and evening. What you eat is far more important than how much you consume.

Another tip to improve your chance for success is to reduce your exposure to the temptations that are always present. Never go to the supermarket when you are hungry. When you do shop for food, avoid areas of the store, such as the bakery and snack section, where high-carbohydrate foods are displayed. Examining the dessert menu in a restaurant and shopping in a bakery are also dangerous activities until your willpower level is well established.

Snacks and nocturnal noshing

For anyone concerned about blood sugar and weight control, the most dangerous hours of the day extend from the end of dinner until bedtime. Most of us spend our evenings at home, surrounded by forbidden temptations of all kinds. In the typical American household, the refrigerator and the pantry shelves hold a cornucopia of carbohydrates in sufficient variety and quantity to send any diabetic into coma. The challenge is to select and consume low-carbohydrate snacks that satisfy your desire to nosh and that won't get you tossed off the wagon.

Here are some tips, that is, things you can do and eat to stay in control:

1. Eat enough at dinner to feel full but not overstuffed.
2. Drink water, zero-carb flavored water, or sugar-free (diet) sodas.
3. Snack on nuts—especially macadamias, peanuts (not honey roasted), Brazil nuts, pecans, walnuts, and cashews.
4. Eat cheese.
5. Prepare and keep handy plenty of low-carbohydrate snacks (hard-boiled eggs, pickles, chopped-up veggies like celery, cucumber, or broccoli, for example).
6. Snack on sugar-free Jell-O, puddings, popsicles, ice cream, etc.
7. Drink commercially available low-carbohydrate protein shakes.
8. Be active instead of sedentary.

Try to make snack portions small and let as much time as possible pass between snacking sessions. For instance, eat a few nuts instead of a handful. If you are active instead of sedentary, you will also snack less. Sitting in front of the television is dangerous (for more than dietary reasons). Schedule activities for yourself and your family that involve personal interaction. If weather permits, try outdoor activities, especially sports, walking, exercise, etc. Sitting promotes consuming food, usually of the sweet, forbidden kind. Activity is healthy on many levels, and you might actually complete chores that have been on your to-do list for months.

Unfortunately, most are always looking for the easy way, a magic pill, to achieve weight loss and good health. Intellectually, we know it doesn't exist, but that doesn't stop us from searching for a painless alternative to get what we want.

While the Five-Finger Lifestyle is close to painless, it does require commitment to a plan of action. As you continue to read this book, you will realize how you can use the Five-Finger Lifestyle to eat pleasurably but wisely and achieve weight loss and blood sugar control.

Today, Tomorrow, and Forever

The intent and design of the Five-Finger Lifestyle diet is to provide you with an outline for a simple, easy-to-follow, no-brainer eating program. From a long-term perspective, however, it is meant to be a foot in the door, just like what a door-to-door salesman does to prevent you from slamming the door in his face. As such, I urge you to commit to follow the Five-Finger Lifestyle strictly for a full two months. During that time, eliminate carbohydrates from your diet to the greatest degree possible. If you are diligent, careful, and faithful, almost all of you will see positive results. You will lose weight. You will feel healthier and have more energy. If you are diabetic, you will experience consistently lower fasting blood sugars, lower hemoglobin A1c results, and a reduction in large fluctuations in blood sugar levels.

That is the foot in the door I am talking about. Success in achieving these goals will encourage you to continue adhering to the low-carbohydrate dietary concept. You will have seen firsthand that limiting carbohydrate intake is a positive and healthy alternative for life.

After your successful first two months, your reward is the ability to experiment with food choices and to increase selections while preserving your commitment to restricting carbohydrate intake. The trick is to eat a greater variety of foods without significantly increasing the amount of carbohydrate you consume.

All carbohydrates in food are not equal. It is possible to eat some carbohydrates but limit or modify their impact on your blood sugar and body weight.

The concept of net carbs is the cornerstone of the Atkins Diet, the low-carbohydrate regimen popularized by Robert C. Atkins, MD. To determine grams of net carbs per serving, subtract the grams of fiber and the grams of sugar alcohols from the total carbohydrate grams. The net carb value of a food indicates its impact on blood sugar and the degree of challenge it presents to the insulin system. This simple mathematic calculation allows you to control the total amount of carbohydrates you consume each day. Since the numbers are low, the math is easy to do in your head. It is also easy to keep track of the grams of carbohydrate consumed throughout the day either mentally or with a small notebook. If a food contains little or no carbs—like meat, cheese, and eggs—you can eat large amounts with no impact on the daily carbohydrate total. Foods that contain carbohydrates with a low net carbohydrate value can be eaten in reasonable quantities. Once you are able to increase your maximum daily carbohydrate target, you have greater flexibility in choosing what to eat.

Some commercially available dietary regimens rely on the concept of the glycemic index. The glycemic index (GI) ranks carbohydrates on a scale of 0 to 100 based on the height and speed of the blood sugar increase after eating. Foods with a high GI are rapidly absorbed and quickly cause significant fluctuations in blood sugars. Low GI foods are absorbed more slowly and have less of an immediate impact on blood sugar levels. Popularly, this is known as fast or bad carbs and slow or good carbs.

The glycemic index is a valid principle that can be used to expand food choices once you have established reliable low-carbohydrate eating habits with the Five-Finger Lifestyle. Foods that produce a gradual rise in blood sugar create less strain on the carbohydrate-insulin system, but it is important to realize that even slow carbs do raise the blood sugar. This fact is especially important for diabetics. In my experience, dietary regimens that rely on glycemic index work better for weight control than for sugar control.

Portion control is, therefore, an important element of glycemic index theory. The term *glycemic load* takes into account both the glycemic index and the actual amount of carbohydrates the portion and the food item contains. Glycemic load is a calculation that is too complex to be used as part of a dietary regimen as it requires a measurement of each portion size. Proponents of the glycemic index suggest combining servings of high GI foods with low GI foods to achieve an average GI level for a meal. This exchange concept is similar to that found in regulated-calorie diets such as those promoted by the American Diabetic Association. The complexity of these diet models makes them difficult for most people to understand and use.

Because the Five-Finger Lifestyle is about simplicity, I prefer to use the net carb concept. The carbohydrate content of any food can be determined using simple subtraction. Your goal is simply to minimize your daily total carbohydrate intake. You don't have to carry a glycemic index chart around with you. Simply read the label, and do the math.

In the expanded phase of the Five-Finger Lifestyle, what you eat is determined primarily by its carbohydrate content and not the size of the portion. This is an important concept. Portion size is relevant only in foods that have significantly higher net carb values. For instance, suppose you plan to eat a 25-gram carbohydrate meal. You choose tuna salad because it has no carbs. One slice of low-carb bread contains 8 grams of carbohydrates. Your choice, therefore, is whether to have an open-faced sandwich (8 grams of carbs) or a traditional sandwich (16 grams of carbs). Obviously, if you take the open-faced option, you have room in that meal for 17 more grams of carbohydrates in some other form without exceeding your goal.

Use the net carb system to augment the variety of food you eat while remaining within your total daily carbohydrate goals. The more you fill up on low-carbohydrate foods, the more space you will have for treats that have a higher net carb value. When purchasing prepared foods, remember that some containers of prepared food may actually contain more than one serving.

Daily carbohydrate consumption goals

Since it is not possible to eliminate carbohydrates totally, it is essential that you establish a daily carbohydrate intake target. The average American eats well over 800 grams of carbohydrates per day, a lot of which are useless carbohydrates. Eating them can be avoided. As such, I should name them discretionary carbohydrates since one chooses to eat them even it is unnecessary to do so. It should be obvious that sodas, candies, fast foods on soft white buns, pastries, doughnuts, sweet packaged snacks, and sugar in your coffee will quickly raise your blood sugar and, therefore, must be eliminated from your diet. There is just no excuse for eating foods that are clearly high in sugar.

During the first two months, limit your carbohydrate intake to between 20 and 40 grams each day. This goal is very important, and you should plan to achieve it. To do so, you will need to use all the rules, suggestions, hints, and tricks we have discussed up to this point. This is the time to strictly eliminate the food groups enumerated on the five fingers of the Five-Finger Lifestyle model.

After your initial and, hopefully, successful two-month adherence to the Five-Finger Lifestyle regimen, you can gradually raise your daily carbohydrate intake. This is not an invitation to precipitously fall off the low-carb wagon. You must still adhere to the principles eliminating the five food group fingers that are high in carbohydrates. Using the simple net carb calculations outlined above, start experimenting with foods at each meal that have slightly higher net carbohydrate content. Set maximum carb intake levels and adhere to them. Most of you will find that a daily net carb intake of about 80 grams is an attainable and reasonable goal. This will allow you a wide variety of taste choices while maintaining your weight and blood sugar numbers in an acceptable range. If your weight or blood sugar starts creeping up, go back to a lower daily net carbohydrate consumption.

This technique of self-monitoring gives you control and responsibility for your own body.

Carb creep, willpower, and self-control

In this book, I have outlined a lifestyle that is simple to follow. It is a lifestyle that I know works from personal experience. It will give you the opportunity to lose weight, control your blood sugar, and still eat many foods that you love including meats and sweets.

But . . .

No matter how you slice it, no eating regimen can be successful without willpower and self-control. Temptation surrounds you in many forms.

Grabbing a bite in a restaurant is so much easier than preparing a meal, especially after working all day. You can mitigate the carbohydrate impact of eating out by choosing low-carbohydrate items from the menu. Most restaurants are now aware of the concept of carbohydrate restriction and will serve sandwiches open-faced and substitute vegetables for potatoes. The more you prepare your own food, however, the more you will appreciate knowing exactly what you are eating and where it comes from.

If you live with others, don't expect them to live the Five-Finger Lifestyle along with you. This puts high-carbohydrate foods within easy reach, in fact right under your nose. Usually these are the comfort foods—the sweet temptations you have been happily eating all your life while your weight and blood sugar have been slowly rising.

This is precisely the point where you must exercise true willpower and self-control. It is so easy to excuse a tiny bite of forbidden pleasure—"It's only one bite. How many carbs could it have?" "I have been doing so well. One bite (meal, snack, day, etc.) off my five-finger lifestyle won't hurt." This is *carb creep*—tiny indiscretions that, if unchecked, add up to enough carbohydrates to destroy your chances for success.

No excuses allowed

I am going to give you a tool to help you out. A number of years ago, I remember seeing a television story about a man who called himself a breathologist. He claimed that he ate absolutely no food at all but sustained himself merely by inhaling molecules of food nasally. I never actually saw a verification of his story, but I remember joking that I wouldn't want to be sitting in front of his refrigerator at 3:00 AM!

Nevertheless, I adopted his technique for myself when it came to forbidden food items. Take a long, slow whiff of that great aroma and imagine having some in your mouth. This really works, and in a group situation, it can actually cause laughter (*with* you, not *at* you). One word of caution—be careful not to drool on someone else's piece.

Bottom line here: You have to want it. You have to commit to it. You must accept the fact that you will forgo some accustomed pleasures. You have to opt *for* weight control, *for* blood sugar control, and *for* better health to succeed. There is no magic potion, no pill, and no program that allows you to eat anything you want and still be slim and healthy.

The Five-Finger Lifestyle gives you a starting place and framework to find both immediate and long-term success without purchasing a home gym and prepared foods you may not like the taste of and without using a scale, calculator, and ruler every time you sit down to eat.

The Five-Finger Lifestyle
Adaptability And Portability

On the surface, you could think that the Five-Finger Lifestyle is overly restrictive and difficult to follow, especially for an extended time. After all, I am asking you to give up foods that you eat every day, foods you have eaten all your life, and foods that you really love to eat. Even if the payoff is weight loss, normal blood sugar levels, and improved health for a longer life, you may not want to give up everything without a fight.

My job is to convince you that the Five-Finger Lifestyle really offers you the simplest and easiest way to achieve success in this most vital and difficult task.

There are several reasons that most of us fail to adhere to dietary regimens:

1. We refuse to stop eating foods we really love.
2. We spend times of inactivity and boredom in the presence of abundant food.
3. We live busy lives that require eating outside the home.
4. We don't establish regular mealtimes, allowing hunger to reach emergency levels with resulting binge feeding.
5. We use numerous excuses to avoid preparation of healthy meals.
6. We lack the willpower and desire to achieve long-term success.

The *adaptability* and *portability* of the Five-Finger Lifestyle is your tool to overcome these obstacles. The Five-Finger Lifestyle is a combination of restriction and permission, and it is my purpose to teach you how to use both to your advantage.

Portability is the ability to follow your eating regimen anytime of the day anywhere in the world. *Adaptability* allows you to substitute food items based on availability and personal tastes.

Here is an example of a situation that frequently arises. You are out shopping with friends or meeting with business associates, and someone says, "Let's grab a bite to eat for lunch in this restaurant." Trust me. It is not a problem for you to eat out with your group and still limit your carbohydrate intake.

When considering what to order, start by avoiding the five foods that are restricted: bread or baked goods, potatoes and root vegetables, rice, pasta, and fruit except for berries. Pass up on the hot bread, garlic rolls, fried noodles, tortilla chips, and assorted crackers that appear on the table. You will have to use some of that willpower. Next, look for protein, vegetables, and dairy products on the menu. Salads are a great choice as they are both low in carbohydrates and healthy. You can make a meal from a salad (no croutons or sweet dressings!) especially if you add protein such as turkey, salmon, or ham.

Choosing a main course that contains mainly protein is usually easy, but the side items are typically high in carbohydrates. Most restaurants are happy to substitute vegetables for potato or rice. If you avoid the high-carbohydrate side items, the incidental carbohydrates used to prepare your main course are generally not significant.

In other words, the thin bread coating on your fish fillet or veal francaise won't put you over your carb limit if you don't eat the rice or twice-baked potato that comes with it.

If your friends have chosen a sandwich shop, you still have good options. You can get any sandwich without bread and use a knife and fork. If being totally different is a problem, try a low-carbohydrate wrap or open-faced sandwich. Both of these options will limit your carbohydrate load. Of course, do not eat the french fries, potato chips, hush puppies, or cookies that come on the side.

Last night, the kids wanted to eat out at a small family-run New York—style pizzeria. Again, this was no problem for me. I started off with a large salad topped with homemade balsamic vinaigrette dressing. To avoid devouring the homemade garlic twists, I inhaled their aroma deeply and used maximum willpower. When the delicious pizza arrived, I scraped all the cheese and meat topping onto my plate and ate it with a knife and fork. At home after dinner, my dogs really enjoyed their pizza-crust treats.

Another aspect of *adaptability* concerns ethnic and preference issues involved with the five restricted food items. Here is where I can demonstrate to you that compromise is an important part of life and of the Five-Finger Lifestyle.

Suppose you are Italian and pasta has always been a significant part of your diet. The Five-Finger Lifestyle tells you to avoid pasta, a high-carbohydrate food. Here is my reasonable compromise.

Last week, I made baked ziti for dinner—one of my family's favorite meals. I made my own thick meat sauce, mixed it with pasta cooked al dente, layered the sauce-pasta mixture with cheeses, and baked the casserole in the oven. I also made garlic-cheese bread sticks and a salad. One serving of that dinner contains enough carbohydrates for several days, so that's not an option for me.

Here's what I did. I set aside a nice portion of that delicious meat sauce. At dinner, I toasted one piece of low-carbohydrate bread, put the sauce on the toast, melted cheese over it all, and ate it with a knife and fork. To satisfy my pasta desire, I had a small portion, about 1-2 tablespoons of the baked ziti. As for the garlic-cheese bread, I had one small bite, just enough to get a taste. For a vegetable, I had cucumbers previously marinated in a Splenda-sweetened vinegar-mayonnaise dressing. In this manner, I was able to participate in our family dinner and enjoy the meal without falling off the low-carb wagon.

Now there are a variety of low-carbohydrate pasta products available. Be sure to read the label carefully—first, to determine what is considered a single serving size and second, to be certain that the calculated carbohydrate content of the serving is accurate. Then, of course, don't eat more than one serving.

Asian cuisine presents another example of the *adaptability* of the Five-Finger Lifestyle. The wok is an incredibly useful tool to prepare meals with a large variety of foods. In Asian cuisine, a marinated fish or meat is stir-fried in ground nut oil (usually peanut oil) with virtually any combination of vegetables, all in a flavorful cooking sauce. Of course, it is customary to serve it over rice. The rice is not essential because you can eat your tasty wok creation on a plate. If you must, have a tablespoon of rice.

Leftovers are one of the greatest benefits of meal preparation. If you make extra dinner, you can have enough food leftover for lunch the next day. Bringing a meal from home avoids the temptations associated with a fast-food or a restaurant lunch. The efficiency of a leftover meal is that you prepare the food only once for two (or more) meals.

It is much easier to control hunger if you eat multiple times during the day. Three main meals make good sense, but hunger gradually increases between meals. Be prepared by taking snacks with you. Don't let your hunger grow until you cannot control the urge to wolf down the first edible thing you see. Invariably, when you are desperately starving, the only food available is a cheese Danish, a glazed doughnut, or a box of Oreos.

By the way, eating a full breakfast is the best way to begin each day. I bet that is just what your mother always told you. Personally, I start each day with two jumbo brown farm eggs—scrambled, fried, or as a cheese omelet, and usually with onions and sausage or bacon. A good breakfast jump-starts your metabolism, giving you the mental and physical energy necessary for work. It also helps you control your morning hunger by avoiding a significant drop in blood sugar.

You have probably heard all this before in various ways and contexts. The Five-Finger Lifestyle is a framework on which to build an eating program that works for each individual.

Diet is a Dirty Word

If I had my way, the word *diet* would be eliminated from the dictionary. To me, a *diet* is something you do for one month before a vacation to look great in a bathing suit. A *diet* is also abandoned on the first day of that vacation. Diets also typically occur as part of New Year's resolutions or immediately after any near-death experience. To most of us, a *diet* is temporary punishment for a life of overindulgence. A *diet* always begins tomorrow or in the morning. In fact, I have even seen diets last as little as sixty seconds!

To be successful with weight control and good diabetic management, we need to make permanent changes in lifestyle. The phrase *lifestyle change* signifies a change of monumental proportions, a volcanic upheaval that sets a person on a totally different pathway forever. It is also a frightening concept to many people. That fear is often used to justify a reluctance to adopt major lifestyle alterations and, once adopted, the inability to follow through over the long haul.

The Five-Finger Lifestyle does require total lifestyle change, nothing less.

Of course, any diet regimen you choose requires the same total commitment. The Five-Finger Lifestyle gives you a simple blueprint to follow so that, once you have made the necessary commitment, you have the highest chance for success.

Understanding Obesity and Diabetes

Diabetes is the leading cause of blindness in the world today. It is also a leading cause of heart attack, stroke, kidney failure, and loss of one's toes and feet. It is a very mean disease. It will leave you blind and crippled in a wheelchair before it kills you.

Obesity puts excessive stress on your heart, making it work harder to circulate blood in your body. It is associated with heart attacks, heart failure, hypertension, arthritis, lack of mobility, and premature death. It is also linked to diabetes, specifically the adult-onset kind.

Like many of our body systems, carbohydrate-insulin balance is automatic. When we eat carbohydrates, the blood sugar level rises. This triggers a release of insulin from specialized islet cells in the pancreas. Insulin helps transport sugar into the cells of the body where it is used for energy. In the normal individual, enough insulin is produced to take care of the elevated blood sugar level, returning it to normal about two hours after eating.

In diabetics, the islet cells do not produce sufficient insulin to bring the blood sugar back down into the normal range. Eating large amounts of carbohydrates challenges the already overtaxed insulin system and causes the blood sugar levels to rise above the normal range. Sugar is a large molecule that cannot cross cell membranes by itself. Elevated blood sugar forces movement of body water from required locations to spaces where it causes organs and cells to malfunction. Both chronically elevated blood sugar and large up-and-down fluctuations in blood sugar are significant risk factors for the development of small blood vessel disease. This characteristic blood vessel pathology of diabetes is responsible for blindness, heart attacks, strokes, and kidney failure.

In general, a patient has to have diabetes for ten to fifteen years before they develop vascular and neurological complications. Sugar control during that first decade, however, will determine to a large degree the severity of these complications and the speed at which they will progress. Two blood tests are currently used to monitor sugar level—fasting blood sugar and the hemoglobin A1c. Fasting blood sugar is the level of blood sugar measured each morning before any food, liquid or solid, is eaten. Numerous devices are commercially available that allow patients to make this measurement at home. The hemoglobin A1c is a measure of average blood sugar levels over several months. Both tests are necessary to assure good diabetic control.

The body needs energy to live. Our metabolism can burn carbohydrates and fats to produce that energy. From an efficiency standpoint, burning carbohydrates is quicker and, therefore, preferred by the cells of our body. To transform fat to energy, a human cell must first convert the fat to sugar. So given a choice, the metabolic processes at the cellular level will choose to burn carbohydrate and store fat for later use. As long as we continue to provide the cell with carbohydrate, fat is stored.

We all know what that looks like.

If a cell doesn't have carbohydrate to burn, however, it must burn fat for energy.

That is the basis of carbohydrate restriction, which changes our metabolism from carbohydrate burning to fat burning. We force the body to use fat instead of storing it. The more we deprive our metabolism of carbohydrate, the more stored fat is used for energy. The result is weight loss and lower blood sugar levels.

When your body burns fat for energy instead of carbohydrate, biochemical compounds called *ketones* are formed. Ketones, an important source of energy for the body, are the natural by-product of fat metabolism.

Michael Eades, MD, has provided this excellent, although somewhat technical, discussion of the role of fat metabolism and ketone formation as part of a low-carbohydrate diet.

Ketones to the rescue.

The liver requires energy to convert the protein to glucose. The energy comes from fat. As the liver breaks down the fat to release its energy to power gluconeogenesis, the conversion of protein to sugar, it produces ketones as a byproduct. And what a byproduct they are. Ketones are basically water soluble (meaning they dissolve in blood) fats that are a source of energy for many tissues including the muscles, brain and heart. In fact, ketones act as a stand in for sugar in the brain. Although ketones can't totally replace all the sugar required by the brain, they can replace a pretty good chunk of it. By reducing the body's need for sugar, less protein is required, allowing the muscle mass (the protein reservoir) to last a lot longer before it is depleted. And ketones are THE preferred fuel for the heart, making that organ operate at about 28 percent greater efficiency.

Fat is the perfect fuel. Part of it provides energy to the liver so that the liver can convert protein to glucose. The unusable part of the fat then converts to ketones, which reduce the need for glucose and spare the muscle in the process.

If, instead of starving, you're following a low-carb diet, it gets even better. The protein you eat is converted to glucose instead of the protein in your muscles. If you keep the carbs low enough so that the liver still has to make some sugar, then you will be in fat-burning mode while maintaining your muscle mass, the best of all worlds. How low is low enough? Well, when the ketosis process is humming along nicely and the brain and other tissues have converted to ketones for fuel, the requirement for glucose drops to about 120-130 gm per day. If you keep your carbs below that at, say, 60 grams per day, you're liver will have to produce at least 60-70 grams of glucose to make up the deficit, so you will generate ketones that entire time.

So, on a low-carb diet you can feast and starve all at the same time. Is it any wonder it's so effective for weight loss?

The Blog of Michael R. Eades, MD
http://www.proteinpower.com/drmike/
Metabolism and Ketosis
May 22, 2007

Medical Aspects of Carbohydrate Restriction

If you are under a physician's care for medical conditions such as diabetes, hypertension, heart disease, or kidney disease, it is essential that you tell your doctor that you plan to use the Five-Finger Lifestyle to lose weight and control your blood sugar. Most likely, he or she will attempt to dissuade you, using some or all of the specious arguments we have covered in previous chapters. At best, be prepared for his outright disapproval. You could try friendly persuasion by buying him his own personal copy of this book.

In the end, however, it is your decision. Once your mind is made up, be firm, open, and frank about your decision with your physician. Emphasize that you are making a lifestyle change that will result in better health. Ask your doctor to support your decision as you will need his help to control the changes that will occur in your body.

If you are a diabetic, your doctor's help is especially important. As your carbohydrate intake decreases, your need for medication to lower your blood sugar may also diminish. Failure to modify your dosage could lead to a serious drop in blood sugar. Your own personal physician or endocrinologist is best equipped to make these adjustments.

Other medical conditions such as hypertension, cardiac disease, arthritis, and lung disease will also benefit from weight loss and sugar control. These conditions rarely change as quickly as blood sugar.

It is also critical to watch your cholesterol levels. While most people on the Five-Finger Lifestyle can tolerate a reasonable quantity of dietary fat, blood cholesterol can rise to unacceptable levels in a small percentage of people. Monitoring the lipid profile, especially during the initial phases of the Five-Finger Lifestyle, is very important. If your cholesterol rises, modification of lipid intake or the use of various lipid-lowering medications may be indicated.

Try to make your doctor an ally in your decision to practice the Five-Finger Lifestyle. Most physicians want their patients to be healthy. It is very frustrating to take care of an endless parade of overweight diabetic patients with out-of-control blood sugars spouting the same excuses. When a patient shows a willingness to make lifestyle changes to become healthier, most doctors will be supportive, especially if there are positive results over time.

About 80 percent of the diabetics I see in my practice are not in good control. A large percentage of my patients, like the population of our country, are also significantly overweight. I discuss weight control and sugar control with all of them and urge them to adopt the Five-Finger Lifestyle. Some are in denial about their condition. Talking to them is like planting a seed in dry ground—it may or may not grow. Most others show some interest, so I spend more time talking with them. Returning patients whom I have converted usually enter the exam room bursting with enthusiasm, eager to tell me how much weight they have lost and how good their sugar levels have been. I always reward these positive achievements by spending even more time talking about food, sharing recipes, and discussing how well they are doing medically.

If you adopt the Five-Finger Lifestyle, lose significant pounds, and control your blood sugar, I am willing to bet that your doctor will be supportive of your efforts, even if he was dead set against your decision initially. Your success will make him a convert.

Serious systemic diseases such as diabetes and hypertension can lead to the collapse of multiple body systems. Kidney failure—a frequent consequence of diabetes—liver failure, and intestinal disorders can cause the body's metabolic functions to become wildly abnormal. Renal dialysis, extraordinary surgical procedures, and very special diets may be necessary to save the patient's life. Under these extreme circumstances, following the Five-Finger Lifestyle may be impossible and even dangerous. Patients in these dire straits should most definitely consult their physician to discuss dietary restrictions.

The role of exercise

Exercise is good for you. In fact, it is essential if you want to maintain cardiac health, muscle tone, overall body strength, mental alertness, good peripheral circulation, and a pleasing appearance. If you want to have the ability to participate successfully and completely in activities that bring you satisfaction and fulfillment, you just cannot spend your life sitting on the couch. Lack of physical activity is undoubtedly related to obesity, poor diabetic control, unhappiness, low self-esteem, joint and muscle maladies, and mental deterioration.

However . . .

Exercise and physical activity are very *inefficient* means to achieve overall weight and sugar control.

For example, look at these numbers:

Calories Burned Related to Exercise
Ref: www.lifelinescreening.com/healthupdates/healthy_you/

Calories burned by 160-pound person in *one hour* when doing the following:

Walking slowly 183
Ballroom dancing 219
Lifting free weights 219
Bicycling at leisurely speed 292
Water aerobics 292

Walking is very important. I urge all my diabetics to walk daily; however, walking for one hour (60 whole minutes) only burns 183 calories. That won't compensate for eating a half-cup serving of rice (380 calories), a cheese Danish (201 calories), or a margarita (219 calories).

The most efficient and effective way to control body weight and blood sugar is supply side restriction. If you don't eat lots of carbohydrates, you won't have to figure out how to remove them from your body.

Muscle cramps

One of the side effects of the Five-Finger Lifestyle is muscle cramps. This is especially true during the initial phase of the lifestyle when carbohydrate restriction is most severe. Although they don't cause permanent damage, leg cramps are painful and can interrupt your sleep.

If you have a cramp, the best treatment is to immediately stretch the muscle. This prevents the muscle fibers from continuing to contract uncontrollably. Frequently, the calf muscle is involved. As soon as the cramp begins, stand on tiptoe to stretch the muscle until the cramp subsides.

Quinine sulfate is usually effective in preventing muscle cramps. Qualaquin is the only quinine compound approved for sale in the USA. Because of potentially serious side effects, it is approved only by prescription for the treatment of malaria. Known risks of quinine therapy include cardiac arrhythmias and thrombocythemia, an elevation in platelet concentration in the blood that can lead to increased risk of blood clots. The FDA banned all over-the-counter quinine compounds in the USA in 1995 and forbids the use of quinine for leg cramps. A variety of quinine sulfate preparations, generic and homeopathic, are available from Canadian pharmacies.

There are alternatives to quinine sulfate that can be used to prevent leg cramps. Tonic water, which contains quinine, is very effective, and sugar-free diet tonic water is available in several brands. Vitamin preparations that contain potassium and magnesium also help as does physical exercise and stretching regimens such as yoga and Pilates.

Dental disease

During childhood and young adult years, finding and treating tooth decay and the cosmetic appearance of your teeth are the principal goals of dental care. In mature individuals, however, the primary cause of dental problems is gum disease. In fact, gum disease is the most common reason for tooth loss in the adult population.

Gum disease is the result of chronic infection in the tissues that surround the roots of the teeth. The infection causes tissue death and bone loss, progressively exposing the root of the tooth. As the resulting "pocket" deepens, the tooth loses its support. Proper gum care—flossing, brushing, and rinsing with medicated solutions—are important preventive measures to save your teeth.

The bacteria that cause gum disease live deep in the "pockets" between the gums and the roots. Like all bacteria, they require carbohydrates to live and grow. Carbohydrate foods, which are chewed and dissolved in the mouth, provide a readily available and abundant source of sugar for these destructive bacteria.

Because the Five-Finger Lifestyle limits the carbohydrate content of the foods you eat, there is a significant reduction in available sugar for the bacteria causing gum disease. To my knowledge, there have been no prospective studies to support this supposition. Anecdotal evidence, however, indicates that a low-carbohydrate diet can help control gum disease and, in some individuals, can even heal diseased gum tissues. Limiting the availability of nutrients for the bacteria that cause gum disease can stop the relentless progression of tissue decay, bone destruction, and subsequent tooth loss.

Low-Carbohydrate Diets:
History And Controversy

We owe an enormous amount of gratitude to Robert C. Atkins, MD, for developing and promoting the concept of the low-carbohydrate diet. The program that bears his name, the Atkins Diet, is a well-conceived eating regimen that has had documented success and is based on solid physiological concepts. For over thirty years, Dr. Atkins and his disciples diligently promoted carbohydrate restriction as a successful alternative to the low-fat, low-calorie diets that were at the time, and still are, the accepted norm.

The concept of carbohydrate restriction was such a departure from conventional thought that vigorous opposition to the Atkins Diet was instantaneous. Critics of the Atkins Diet make two primary claims:

1. The diet is not successful in terms of weight loss and blood sugar control.
2. High-protein, low-carbohydrate diets are dangerous.

In a recent clinical study at Stanford University Medical School, published in *JAMA*, 311 overweight/obese premenopausal women were randomly assigned to follow the Atkins, Zone, LEARN, or Ornish diets. It is important to review here the design, results, and conclusions reached in this landmark study.

OUTCOME MEASURES: Weight loss at 12 months was the primary outcome. Secondary outcomes included lipid profile (low-density lipoprotein, high-density lipoprotein, and non-high-density lipoprotein cholesterol, and triglyceride levels), percentage of body fat, waist-hip ratio, fasting insulin and glucose levels, and blood pressure.

RESULTS: Weight loss was greater (by a factor of 2 times) for women in the Atkins diet group compared with the other diet groups at 12 months. Secondary outcomes for the Atkins group were comparable with or more favorable than the other diet groups.

CONCLUSIONS: In this study, premenopausal overweight and obese women assigned to follow the Atkins diet, which had the lowest carbohydrate intake, lost more weight and experienced more favorable overall metabolic effects at 12 months than women assigned to follow the Zone, Ornish, or LEARN diets. While questions remain about long-term effects and mechanisms, a low-carbohydrate, high-protein, high-fat diet may be considered a feasible alternative recommendation for weight loss.

Gardner CD, Kiazand A, Alhassan S, Kim S, Stafford RS, Balise RR, Kraemer HC, King AC.
JAMA Mar 7 (2007): 297 (9):969-77

These results confirm my own experience, both personal and with my patients. Restricting carbohydrate intake results in weight loss and normalization of blood sugar levels.

Critics cite several purported health risks of low-carbohydrate, high-protein/fat diets.

1. Colon cancer rates are significantly higher in countries whose inhabitants eat a diet high in animal protein, specifically red meat (beef, pork, lamb). General population studies, however, do not take into account the many other epidemiological factors that affect the incidence of specific diseases in large populations. In addition, there are no studies in long-term adherents of Atkins-type diets that demonstrate an increased risk of colon cancer. Although colon cancer is common and lethal, precancerous colon polyps tend to be slow growing. For this reason, the availability and preventive success of colonoscopy can mitigate this potential hazard.

2. Dietary fat consumption, specifically saturated fats and cholesterol, are believed to increase the risk of coronary artery disease. While elevated cholesterol and LDLs (bad cholesterol) are linked to an increased risk of coronary artery disease, it is generally accepted that serum lipid levels in any individual are a product of many factors, not just dietary. Several studies on people using Atkins-type diets at Duke University showed favorable effects on serum lipid levels in the majority of participants (twenty-nine of forty-one in one study). Detractors usually downplay the positive results, highlighting instead the few cases in which cholesterol and LDL levels rose significantly or claiming weight loss alone is responsible for cholesterol lowering. Because lipid metabolism is so person specific, everyone living the Five-Finger Lifestyle should check blood lipid levels periodically. It would be wise to check your blood lipids within one month of starting the Five-Finger Lifestyle and less frequently thereafter as long as the levels remain within normal limits. Lipid concentration may rise, however, in the face of acceptable weight loss and blood sugar levels precisely because diet is not the only factor that influences blood levels of cholesterol and LDLs. There are a variety of over-the-counter and/or prescription medications that can be used to control this problem.

3. Detractors of low-carbohydrate, high-protein diets often raise the prediction of kidney failure from eating large amounts of animal protein. To date, however, there have been no medical studies that demonstrate this to be true.

4. Low-carbohydrate, high-protein diets are somewhat deficient in certain vitamins. Satisfactory vitamin supplements are readily available and should be taken daily, probably by everyone regardless of dietary preferences.
5. There is some indication that high-protein diets lead to increased calcium loss through the kidney. Again, calcium supplements are readily available and should be taken as a preventative for osteoporosis.

Statistics and studies

In our society today, we are bombarded by statistics generated by an army of "professionals" whose goal is to influence and alter our beliefs and behavior. It is difficult, if not impossible, to separate truth from supposition. Study plan, inherent bias by the designer, prejudice of the sponsor, and the inability to factor in all variables usually make the outcomes open to interpretation. Epidemiological population studies can reveal general disease risks, but they are not able to take into account the factors that allow disease to occur in some at-risk individuals and not in others. The incidence of a disease in a population in which a specific risk factor is present does not guarantee causation. It is often cited that Asians living in Asian countries are generally thin despite eating large quantities of rice, a high-carbohydrate food. The implication is that a high-carbohydrate diet does not cause obesity, even though no basis for that conclusion appears in the data. There are obviously many other factors that could be associated with lack of obesity in Asians living in Asia. Since these factors were not studied or discussed, the implied conclusion is not valid.

In many epidemiological studies, coexistence of factors is a common tool used to mislead by implication. It's sort of a birds-of-a-feather type of argument. Using this false logic, I could state that milk is a gateway drug since over 99 percent of all cocaine addicts drank milk as infants. It is equally ridiculous to imply that the predominance of low body weight in Asians eating a high-carbohydrate rice diet proves that low-carbohydrate diets don't work.

An additional difficulty with diet studies in general is the real problem of assessing compliance. The only way to have total control over food intake is for study participants to live full time (24-7) in a clinical center. This ideal design might be possible for a small group of people over a short period. It would not be feasible, however, to "incarcerate" a large enough group of people for a long-enough time to get a statistically valid data sample.

Although anecdotal evidence is not acceptable scientifically, most physicians have a good sense about what therapies are successful for their patients. My experience with carbohydrate restriction has been largely positive. Diabetic patients generally can lose weight, stabilize blood sugar levels, and often decrease or eliminate diabetic medication with the Five-Finger Lifestyle. These goals are especially important in patients with diabetes. Blood sugar control is essential to lessen the risk of diabetic vascular complications such as blindness, heart disease, and amputations. Weight control is also an important part of good general health and a major positive factor in prevention of cardiac disease and hypertension.

Commitment and willpower are required to make lifestyle changes. The Five-Finger Lifestyle provides a framework that is easy to understand and follow. Regardless of its simplicity and adaptability, some don't have the willpower to maintain a low-carbohydrate regimen over the long term. Those that do, however, can expect to maintain better health for a lifetime.

The Politics of Weight Loss

In November 2007, the newspaper *USA TODAY* ran a series of articles concerning obesity and diabetes mellitus. The omission of any useful discussion in the articles about carbohydrate restriction prompted me to write a letter to the editor outlining my Five-Finger Diet for diabetes and weight control.

Simple Diets Work Best with Diabetes

As an ophthalmologist, I treat eye problems in diabetic patients. Diabetes is the leading cause of blindness in the world today ("Diabetes 'revolution' is cutting both ways," Cover story, News, Nov.12).

In numerous studies, elevated blood sugars have been linked to diabetic vision loss despite potentially successful medical and surgical treatments.

Mediation should be used to control blood sugar only after an optimum diet and exercise regimen has been established. Most patients, however, expect medication to control blood sugars no matter what they eat.

They adjust insulin or pill dosages to cover their dietary indiscretions. Unfortunately, dieticians routinely give patients complex diets that require a ruler, a scale and a calculator. It is no wonder that few diabetics can adhere to these elaborate eating regimens.

I explain to my patients that eating carbohydrates is like putting diesel fuel in a vehicle that can only run on gasoline.

Just as a gas engine won't burn diesel, a diabetic's "engine" cannot burn carbohydrates.

I then offer them a simple, five-finger diabetic diet saying: "There are five things you cannot eat: bread and baked goods, potatoes and root vegetables, rice, pasta and fruit except for berries."

Patients who eliminate these items lose weight and can easily control their sugar levels. Expecting patients to abide by a diet that is difficult to follow causes non-compliance and increases their risk of blindness.

Dan Eichenbaum, MD
Murphy, NC

Within a week, two "official" letters were published in *USA TODAY* criticizing the contents of my letter and promoting the agenda of these two groups.

From the American Dietetic Association:

USA TODAY reader Dan Eichenbaum misstates the valuable role that registered dietitians have in helping people with diabetes successfully manage their condition ("Simple diets work best with diabetes," Nov.26).

I regret any negative experiences he or his patients might have had. But a registered dietitian is a crucial part of any diabetic's health care team. Medicare and increasing numbers of private insurance plans recognize this fact by reimbursing the cost of medical nutrition therapy services. Many plans specify registered dietitians as the preferred provider of these potentially lifesaving nutrition services.

Dieticians do not simply hand a person a menu. A registered dietitian takes into account a person's age, weight, blood cholesterol levels and other medical needs to develop a plan that is right for that person.

There is no "one-size-fits-all" eating plan for managing diabetes. Patients need to pay attention to portion sizes, timing of meals and specific food choices. They need to eat smart, avoid weight gain and balance the day's food choices with regular physical activity.

A registered dietitian is the best source of advice in all these areas.

Registered dieticians not only are more educated about the science of food and nutrition than any other health care professional, but they also know how to translate that science into useful, practical advice that anyone can understand and follow.

So, while diabetes can be complex to manage, people with diabetes should know they are not alone.

Connie B. Diekman, president
American Dietetic Association
Chicago

From the American Association of Diabetes Educators:

In his letter to the editor, ophthalmologist Dan Eichenbaum correctly asserts that uncontrolled blood sugar can lead to debilitating complications with diabetes, such as blindness and amputations. But he is mistaken that diabetics should avoid carbohydrates.

By touting his "five-fingered diabetic diet" as the key to weight loss and controlled blood glucose, he is perpetuating misinformation and doing his patients a disservice. Eichenbaum advises patients to avoid "bread and baked goods, potatoes and root vegetables, rice, pasta and fruit except for berries." But that diet severely restricts meal plan options, ignores cultural preferences and lifestyles needs, and often results in increased non-compliance.

Dietitians and diabetes educators stress the necessity of dietary changes and physical activity. Instead of making broad dietary directives that eliminate entire food groups, however, they encourage moderation and reduced portion sizes. They also make dietary recommendations that factor in an individual's cultural tastes and lifestyle requirements.

Diabetes education helps people incorporate behavior change into their lives by personalizing recommendations and simplifying nutritional messages. One example of a simple method for choosing healthy foods for diabetes is the Idaho Plate Method, which suggests filling half a plate with vegetables, a fourth of the plate with bread/ starches and a fourth with lean meat/protein, and having a glass of low-fat milk and a serving of fruit on the side.

There is no simple formula for success with diabetes. Even so, proper education can help a person with diabetes live a full, active life.

Lana Vukovljak, Chief Executive Officer
American Association of Diabetes Educators
Chicago

What lessons can we learn from the two letters written in response to my initial letter? Let's take a look at the content and underlying messages.

The first letter from Connie B. Diekman, president of the American Dietetic Association, makes no secret of her position. At the outset, she states that "*USA TODAY* reader Dan Eichenbaum misstates the valuable role that registered dietitians have in helping people with diabetes." She goes on to assert, "A registered dietitian is the best source of advice in all these areas. Registered dieticians not only are more educated about the science of food and nutrition than any other health care professional, but they also know how to translate that science into useful, practical advice that anyone can understand and follow."

Lana Vukovljak, chief executive officer of the American Association of Diabetes Educators, is concerned about "ignoring cultural preferences and lifestyle needs" and about my "making broad dietary directives that eliminate entire food groups." She tells us that registered dieticians and diabetic educators "encourage moderation and reduced portion sizes [and] also make dietary recommendations that factor in an individual's cultural tastes and lifestyle requirements." She feels I am mistaken in stating that diabetics should avoid carbohydrates. At least she acknowledges that "uncontrolled blood sugar can lead to debilitating complications with diabetes, such as blindness and amputations."

Unfortunately, the common thread of these two letters is turf protection. Both writers lose sight of the real target—weight and blood sugar control—and how to achieve these goals in the general population.

The failures of traditional diet programs over the past forty years are a clear indication that new initiatives are required. Obesity and adult-onset diabetes are increasing in epidemic proportions despite the best efforts of those who offer traditional weight and sugar-control regimens. The facts just don't support anything close to a claim of success. If you need convincing, do some people watching at an airport, city street, or a school.

I have spent over thirty years taking care of patients, talking with them, and helping them remain sighted despite their age and disease. It is not a question of competence of the educators. The problem is that traditional regimens are not practical for average people. Patients cannot fit these complex programs into their personal lives.

Everyone cannot understand and follow traditional ADA diabetic diets. If they could, don't you think more people would be successful at it? My patients assure me that the diet brochures they have received are written in a foreign language even after one-on-one lessons with a dietician. I know some carpenters who are pretty good at eyeballing portion sizes in inches, but most people won't serve themselves a portion using a tape measure. The slicer in the deli probably can estimate weight pretty well, but few of us would expect to use a scale to weigh food at the dinner table. In addition, it is unlikely that any of us would carry a scale, tape measure, and calculator around for when we go out to eat in a restaurant.

In addition, I have yet to find any "exchanges" on the shelves of my local supermarket. When I ask my patients about "exchanges," I usually get the what-planet-are-you-from look.

In the typical patient's hands, portion control is, at best, an approximate quantity. In practice, servings of foods we really like are usually more generously estimated. Put bluntly, for most of us, it would require a larger plate to hold a two-inch square section of apple pie than a two-inch square piece of grilled liver.

It is also inconceivable to me that diabetics and overweight people shouldn't be told to avoid carbohydrates. Diabetes is a disease characterized by the body's inability to handle a carbohydrate load. In fact, the presence of the disease is demonstrated by a significantly elevated blood sugar following a carbohydrate challenge (glucose tolerance test).

It is a fact that chronically elevated blood sugars as well as wide fluctuations in sugar levels are detrimental and lead to the vascular complications that cause disability and death in diabetics. This instability and elevation of blood sugars result directly from eating carbohydrates. So how can you tell a diabetic it is all right to eat a bowl of spaghetti when he would be better off just eating the meat sauce by itself or over a grilled chicken breast? Why counsel an overweight patient to eat baked potatoes or french fries when suitable low-carbohydrate alternatives are preferable and available?

To combat obesity in children, schools are removing regular soda and sugar-filled snacks and foods from on-campus vending machines. This initiative is being undertaken in clear recognition that a diet high in sugars leads to undesirable weight gain. As such, it should also be obvious that carbohydrate restriction on a larger scale, like that recommended by the Five-Finger Lifestyle, would also result in significant weight loss and lower blood sugars.

Carbohydrate restriction is the logical alternative for weight and blood sugar control. The Five-Finger Lifestyle provides both a simple plan to begin living low carb and a solid framework for long-term success.

This book and my unpublished rebuttal letter to *USA TODAY* clearly state and support the case for carbohydrate restriction and the Five-Finger Lifestyle.

I read with interest the two rebuttal letters in yesterday's USA TODAY from Ms. Dickman of the American Dietetic Association and Lana Vukovljak of the American Association of Diabetic Educators (USA TODAY, December 5).

Frankly, I am not surprised by the content of their letters. As a well-trained physician, I recognize that a multifaceted lifestyle modification is required to control both obesity and diabetes. Unfortunately, the ADA and the AADE, as well as many other organizations, have spent decades trying to bring about that change using complex diet regimens and often-conflicting advice.

A constant parade of overweight patients and out-of-control diabetics in my office and in physician's offices everywhere is testimony to the fact that these complicated programs just do not work for the vast majority of patients.

As the Chinese proverb instructs, "A journey of a thousand miles begins with a single step." The Five Finger Lifestyle Diet I outlined in my letter is just that—a simple beginning step for patients to control their weight and blood sugar. Once a patient experiences personal results, i.e., weight loss and sugar control, it is easier to accept other necessary aspects of a healthy lifestyle such as exercise and a more personalized dietary regimen.

After decades of failure, new incentives must be offered to address our national epidemic of obesity and adult-onset diabetes. A simple diet plan that provides short-term good results without burdensome compliance standards is a better incentive for average individuals to achieve long term personal success.

Dan Eichenbaum, MD
Murphy, NC

Low-Carbohydrate Cooking at Home

It is not my intention to create or provide an extensive low-carbohydrate cookbook. Instead, I will provide you some recipes that are illustrative of how to prepare interesting and tasty home-cooked meals that fall within the guidelines I have given you in this book. For me, inventing new and unique low-carbohydrate recipes through experimentation is the most enjoyable challenge of following the Five-Finger Lifestyle.

We have already discussed how to determine the carbohydrate content of various foods and recipe components. Now is the time to use all your skills to become the creative low-carbohydrate chef that is hiding within each of you.

The first group of recipes (wok cooking, low-carb pizza, and skillet fry) are provided to illustrate how to start with a simple, basic cooking style and then modify the ingredients to achieve a variety of taste choices to avoid monotony.

Cooking with a Wok

I find that cooking in the Asian style using a wok allows for incredible flexibility and unlimited creativity. Five basic components are used in a mix-and-match fashion:

1. Protein source: beef, pork, chicken, scallops, shrimp, and tofu are the most commonly used, but any meat or meat alternative in any form or cut can be used.

2. Vegetables: most commonly used are onions, cabbage, string beans, snow peas, celery, peppers, carrots, and broccoli, but almost any vegetable can be used depending on your particular tastes and carbohydrate content.
3. Marinade: the protein source is generally marinated prior to cooking to infuse a flavor of choice.
4. Cooking sauce: this is a sauce used at the end of the cooking process to provide an overall flavor to the dish—to tie in all the individual tastes under one umbrella, so to speak.
5. Spices and miscellaneous embellishments: salt, pepper, and garlic are spices we usually use, but Asian cuisine uses a variety of additional spices (such as ginger, sesame, or curry) to achieve characteristic tastes.

Once you choose the ingredients, the next step is preparation of the components. Some phases of the cooking process proceed rapidly and others more slowly. For this reason, prepare all components of your dish first. If you do all the chopping, cutting, and sauce making in advance, the actual cooking process will proceed smoothly with less anxiety on the part of the chef.

1. Protein source: Beef, pork, and chicken are usually either cut into small chunks, shaved very thin, or cut into strips. Shrimp and scallops are usually left whole. When using tofu, select the firmest product available so that it will stay intact when being cooked.
2. Vegetables: vegetables may be thinly sliced, shaved, or used in chunks depending on the consistency of the item.
3. Marinade: The choices here are endless and depend on the taste you are trying to achieve. Because the marinade is primarily for the protein source, it usually is more simple and is tailored to complement the particular meat to be used.
4. Cooking sauce: Again, you have great latitude here. Since the cooking sauce applies to the entire creation, it is generally more complex and made up of a larger variety of items
5. Spices and miscellaneous embellishments: Use spices to augment the overall taste, not overpower it. For example, soy sauce can have significant salt content. If you also add table salt, the final result may be overly salty. Dry-roasted peanuts chopped into a coarse powder, sesame seeds, or roasted cashews can be added at the end of the cooking process or just before serving to enhance the appearance and taste.

Now for the rules of wok cooking:

1. Always preheat the wok using medium-high heat. You are ready to cook when the top edge of the wok is too hot to touch.
2. Use peanut oil. It won't burn with high heat used in wok cooking.
3. Generally, the first item in the wok is chopped onions. A clove or two of crushed garlic up front is also a good idea.
4. Add items based on estimated cooking time. The protein source generally takes the longest to cook, so add it first (after the onions and garlic). Add vegetables once the meat is fully cooked. Harder vegetables and bigger chunks of vegetables (carrots and celery) should be added before soft vegetables like green onions and cabbage.
5. Once all items are cooked, push items to the side, leaving the center of the wok without food. Pour the cooking sauce into this center "pit" and stir while the sauce thickens. Once it starts to thicken, mix in the meat and vegetables.
6. Top with garnish like sesame seeds, etc.
7. If you like your Asian meal spicy, add ground fresh chili paste (*sambal oelek*) or cook a few chili peppers in with the food.
8. It is, of course, customary to eat Asian food with rice, which you cannot do as part of a low-carbohydrate lifestyle. Low-carbohydrate pasta (Dreamfields), however, is now commercially available and is an excellent substitute for rice. Precook the pasta until it is al dente, drain, and butter it. You can serve your dish over the pasta or put the pasta into the wok with the cooked meal just before serving.

Here are some suggestions for the marinades and cooking sauces:

Simple Marinade (for 1 Pound of Meat)

Mix the following in a bowl and then pour over prechopped meat or other protein source:

2 tablespoons of sherry or cooking wine
1 or 2 teaspoons of corn starch
1 clove of crushed garlic

Cooking Sauce

Mix the following in a bowl and save for cooking:

> 1 tablespoon of sherry or cooking wine
> 2 tablespoons of soy sauce
> 2 teaspoons of sesame oil
> 1 or 2 teaspoons of cornstarch

Indonesian-Style Cooking Sauce

Mix the following in a bowl and heat on a low flame:

> 1 tablespoon of sherry or cooking wine
> 2 tablespoons of soy sauce with ginger
> 2 teaspoons of sesame oil

Stir in 1 tablespoon of peanut butter to the heated mixture.
Remove from the heat when the peanut butter is dissolved and the sauce is smooth.
Stir in 1 or 2 teaspoons of cornstarch as the sauce is cooling.
The essence of Asian cooking is experimentation. Have fun!

Low-carbohydrate pizza

> Crust
> Hamburger (lean) 0.5 pound
> Ground pork 0.5 pound
> Italian spices to taste

Mix well and pat as thin as possible on the bottom of a pie dish or cookie sheet with sides to contain the grease.
Bake for 15 minutes at 425 degrees. Pour out the grease.

Topping

Spread over the crust a thin layer of commercial pizza sauce, or make your own with tomato paste, water, olive oil, and garlic.

Add whatever toppings you want and lots of shredded cheese.
Bake at 425 degrees for about 12 minutes or until the cheese melts and starts to bubble.
Let it cool a bit, slice, and eat.

Skillet fry

Skillet fry is similar to wok cooking in that a variety of protein sources and vegetables are used with spices to make a meal. I use skillet fry, however, to prepare meals that are more European style in taste. Here is a sample recipe to use as a template:

1. Cut boneless, skinless chicken breasts into chunks and season with celery salt, paprika, Italian spices, and coarse ground pepper. Soak in heavy cream.
2. Precook low-carbohydrate pasta al dente in water seasoned with a chicken bouillon for flavor. Drain pasta. Melt butter in the pasta pot, and return pasta to the pot. Flavor it with pepper and grated parmesan cheese. Set it aside.
3. Heat the skillet. Melt butter in it and add some olive oil. Sauté chopped onions and garlic, then drain chicken and add it to the skillet. Cook chicken pieces thoroughly, turning frequently. If you have room in your carbohydrate total, consider adding a small amount of flavored bread crumbs (1/3 cup generally has about 18 grams of carbs).
4. As cooking the chicken nears completion, add whatever vegetables you have already chopped.
5. Add the prepared pasta and mix well. Top with shaken parmesan cheese.

Dr Dan's Pizza Dip

INGREDIENTS

> Cream Cheese 8 oz
> Ground Beef 1 lb
> Pizza Sauce 14 oz
> Red Onion Half medium sized, chopped
> Mushrooms chopped
> Pepperoni about ½ lb sliced thin and chopped
> Pizza Cheese one 8-oz package finely shredded

PIZZA FILLING

Saute onions in butter. When clarified, add ground beef and cook well, seasoning with Italian seasonings and coarse-ground black pepper. When meat is near done, add in the mushrooms and the pepperoni. Drain of grease and add pizza sauce. Cook until all ingredients are well blended together.

THE DIP

In a 10" glass pie plate, spread softened cream cheese to cover the bottom
Put Pizza Filling in next
Cover entire top with finely shredded Pizza Cheese mix
Bake uncovered at 350 for 25-30 minutes (until cheese is well melted)
Serve warm with chips, in a bowl, etc

Dr Dan's Salsa Dip

> Cream Cheese 8 oz
> Dr Dan's Taco Meat 1 lb ground beef (see recipe below)
> Salsa Mild one 8 oz jar
> Shredded Mexican Cheese 1 package

Taco Meat

Chop half a White Onion and saute in butter; coarse ground black pepper and Adobo seasoning to taste

Add 1 lb Ground Chuck or Round-cook until done; drain grease

On low heat, add 1 package taco seasoning and 1/3 cup of water. Stir well so meat is well coated with seasoning.

Add finely chopped Cilantro (about ½ a bunch)

The Dip

In a 10" pie pan, spread softened cream cheese to cover the bottom of the pie plate

Put Taco Meat mixture in next

Put Salsa in next

Cover entire top with finely shredded Mexican Cheese mix

Bake uncovered at 350 for 25-30 minutes (until cheese is well melted)

Serve warm with chips, in a bowl with lettuce, wrapped in a taco, etc

HALF SOUR PICKLES

From my mother

> 4 tsp. Kosher coarse salt
> 6 cucumbers
> 3-4 stalks celery
> 1 med. onion, sliced
> 2 lg. garlic cloves, crushed
> 1/2 cup vinegar
> 1 cup water

Mix salt, vinegar and water in a 2—Quart glass measuring cup. Be sure salt dissolves completely. Slice cucumbers along their length and pack 1/2 of the slices along with celery, garlic and onion into a 1-Quart Mason jar. It is easier to use a wide mouth jar. Finish packing the jar with the remainder of the cucumber slices (jar will be tightly packed). Pour the salt-vinegar-water mixture into the Mason jar, filling it to the brim. Top off jar with water if necessary, tightly cover, and refrigerate for 1 week before using.

It is also possible to vary this recipe based on your needs. You can make the pickling marinade with water, vinegar, garlic, salt, celery salt, and onion and put in any sealable container. Cut up cucumbers or any other vegetables such as carrots or celery and put in the container, seal it, and put in the refrigerator. After a week or two, it is ready to eat. You can actually refill the container with freshly cut vegetables several times before the marinade needs to be re-made.

SWEET STUFF

Most of us get into trouble from a carbohydrate point of view because of the sweet tooth your mom gave you. There are, of course, commercially available sugar-free snacks you can buy from the store. Be careful with this! Some items are low in carbohydrate content, but the serving size is small, and there is more than one serving in the container. You are fine with the first serving, but the temptation to keep eating will break the carbohydrate meter. There are some sugar-free gelatins, yogurts, and puddings that are truly low in carbohydrate content. Again, it is tough to stop at just one.

There are, however, some delicious homemade treats and tricks you can use to satisfy the craving for sweets without breaking the carbohydrate bank in the process.

Here are a few suggestions:

Sweetened Berry Bowl

Strawberries, raspberries, and blueberries make a great sweet treat. Wash the berries first, then cut the strawberries into thin slices. Put all the berries into a sealable container, cover with Splenda, cover the container, and shake it so that the Splenda mixes well with the berries. Put in the refrigerator for a few days so that a natural sauce will form. Eat with whipped cream, or pour over low-carbohydrate ice cream.

Low-Carbohydrate Cheesecake

Most of the ingredients in a cheesecake are low in carbohydrates. It's the sugar that gets you. Despite claims to the contrary, artificial sweeteners will bake off, so the standard cheesecake recipes with eggs do not result in a satisfactory product.

I suggest you begin with a basic recipe for cheesecake that does not require baking—cream cheese, whipped cream, vanilla, and Splenda. From that point, I can choose any number of flavor options—sugar-free caramel, sugar-free chocolate, sugar-free Amaretto, sugar-free hazelnut, lemon juice, key lime juice, or berries from the sweetened berry bowl for example.

So how do we put it all together?

Pie Crust

If you are well along the low-carbohydrate trail, you can use commercially available graham cracker powder to make a pie crust. By my calculation, using the recipe on the box with two tablespoons of cinnamon-sugar mix instead of sugar, the total carbohydrate content of a graham cracker crust is about 100 grams for the entire crust or (cut into 10 pieces) about 10 grams per slice of pie.

> Graham cracker crumbs 1.25 cup
> Cinnamon-sugar 2 tablespoons
> Butter 1/3 cup or 5.33 tablespoons

Dry mix graham cracker crumbs and cinnamon-sugar well.
Melt butter and add to above mixture.
Mix well with clean hands.
Spray an 8-inch glass pie plate with PAM.
Put the graham cracker mixture into plate and push flat and up the sides.
Bake at 325 degrees for 8 minutes. Remove from oven and let cool completely.

A pie crust made from pecans is a lower carbohydrate alternative.

Pie Crust from Pecans

> Crushed pecans 1.25 cup
> Melted butter 2/3 cup
> Splenda or Splenda baking mixture 0.5 cup
> Cinnamon several teaspoons

Pecans—whole, finely chopped, or powdered—are commercially available. Of course, you can buy whole nuts and grind them to a powder yourself. Try to purchase pecans that have an equal amount of carbohydrate and fiber (e.g., carbohydrate, 4 grams; fiber, 3-4 grams). That will give you 1 gram or less of carbs per serving and lower the overall carbohydrate content of the crust.

Directions

1. Chop/crush pecans as fine as possible, or for best results, purchase pecans that are already crushed into a fine powder.
2. Add Splenda and cinnamon powder.
3. Add melted butter and mix into a paste.
4. Form pecan paste to bottom (and sides if desired) of an 8-inch pie plate or springform pan.
5. Bake at 325 degrees until crust is firm (a maximum of 8 minutes or less).
6. Let cool before putting in filling.

Cheesecake Filling (Basic Recipe)

> Cream cheese 2 8-ounce packages at room temperature
> Vanilla extract 1 tablespoon
> Splenda (granulated) 1.5 to 2 cups
> Whipped cream 4-8 ounces (more or less to get desired consistency)

Some suggested flavorings to add (amount added to achieve desired taste):

1. Caramel syrup (sugar free)
2. Key lime juice (unsweetened)
3. Chocolate syrup (sugar free)
4. Lemon juice
5. Sweetened berry bowl
6. Sugar-free syrups such as hazelnut, Amaretto, Grand Marnier, etc.
7. Baked apple: line crust with pieces before adding filling (great with caramel)

Procedure

1. Use an electric mixer.
2. Add ingredients one at a time in the above order with the mixer running at moderately slow speed.
3. Once all the ingredients are added, beat at more rapid speed to blend well.
4. Spoon into cooled pie crust (above).
5. Chill.
6. To serve, put whipped cream around the rim.
7. Decorate with sugar-free chocolate, caramel, Melba sauce (below), etc.

Raspberry (Melba) Sauce

Ingredients

Red and/or black raspberries 2 pounds
Water 4 tablespoons
Splenda 3 cups
Grand Marnier (optional) 1-3 tablespoons
Cornstarch 1 tablespoon premixed in 1 tablespoon of water

Directions

1. Simmer berries with 4 tablespoons of water in saucepan until mixture turns to mush.
2. Strain through a fine-mesh strainer. Keep the *juice* and discard the *seeds.*
3. Put the juice back into the saucepan and heat on low flame.
4. Add Grand Marnier (optional).
5. Add Splenda and stir until it dissolves.
6. Bring to a light boil and add cornstarch liquid and stir to thicken.
7. Turn off flame, cool, and store in refrigerator.

Use to top cheesecake, ice cream, or fruit.

Baked Apple

Ingredients

Apples 2 firm, fresh apples
Butter 1 tablespoon
Brown sugar 1 tablespoon (12-gram carbs)
Cinnamon 1 teaspoon
Caramel syrup (sugar free) 1 tablespoon
Water 0.5 cup

Procedure

1. Melt butter.
2. Add brown sugar, cinnamon, caramel syrup, and water and heat until smooth.
3. Peel and core the apple. If you can, slice apples horizontally into rings, restack, and put into baking dish.
4. Preheat oven to 350 degrees.
5. Pour liquid mixture over apples into baking dish.
6. Bake for about 1 hour until soft, basting apples frequently with liquid mixture.

The Five-Finger Lifestyle Club

I don't know who invented the term *support group*. It's a great strategy for achieving success, especially when you are trying to do something new or difficult. Humans are social animals and derive comfort from others who are struggling with similar problems. In addition, it is not surprising that the odds of success improve significantly when you participate in a group effort. By forming your own personal support group to live the Five-Finger Lifestyle, you become surrounded by people whose eating habits are the same as your own. You will have lots to talk about, such as food choices and recipes. Controlling temptation is also easier when you can share the risk with others in your group.

Your support group should consist of people with whom you spend lots of time. Generally, that would be your colleagues at work and your family. Although you spend a significant portion of your waking hours on the job, meal-eating time is usually limited. Finding people with whom you are socially and "dietetically" compatible, however, is not difficult, especially if you have a large-enough group from which to choose. Most people claim to be on a diet much of the time, even if they plan to start next Monday. This is especially true before and after holidays, summertime, and vacations. Make plans to eat meals with your Five-Finger Lifestyle club members. Arrange snack time as a group as well, and above all, don't keep snacks at your desk or workstation.

At home, forming a like-minded eating group may be more difficult. For one, your choices are limited to family members living with you (i.e., a smaller group than at work). Your kids (if you have them and they live with you) will probably have their own ideas about proper eating habits, which will not consist of eliminating french fries, pizza, sandwiches, and pasta. If members of an older generation (like parents and grandparents) live with you, changing their ideas about what constitutes a good meal will probably be nearly impossible. Most likely, it will be your spouse and you against the world—a great way to fortify your relationship. Worst-case scenario, you may have to become a gastronomic army of one.

In writing this book and preparing it for publication, I asked several coworkers, employees, nurses, and friends to read a rough draft and try living the Five-Finger Lifestyle as outlined. Others heard about the project and asked to be included. They all became charter members of my own Five-Finger Lifestyle Club. Discussing our successes and techniques became a daily routine. Soon we were also sharing recipes, many of which appear in this book. The spontaneous and unspoken challenge was to achieve the best-tasting, most-satisfying delicacy with the lowest number of carbohydrates (i.e., the best taste-per-carb ratio).

I encourage you all to do the same. It will increase your success and help you achieve your weight loss and sugar control objectives.